All Homemade Beauty Products

Easy to Make Body Lotions and Creams, Scrubs and Body Butters Recipes

Josephine Simon

Body wrap. w/loss

1) Full Body Scrub + brush

2) ginger powder 2 tsp ↑

   5 tps Betonite clay

   10 tsp watm water 20-30 mins

DISCLAIMER

All rights reserved. No part of this publication or the information in it may be quoted from or reproduced in any form by means such as printing, scanning, photocopying, or otherwise without prior written permission of the copyright holder.

Disclaimer and Terms of Use: Effort has been made to ensure that the information in this book is accurate and complete. However, the author and the publisher do not warrant the accuracy of the information, text, and graphics contained within the book due to the rapidly changing nature of science, research, known and unknown facts, and internet. The author and the publisher do not hold any responsibility for errors, omissions, or contrary interpretation of the subject matter herein. This book is presented solely for motivational and informational purposes only. The publisher and author of this book does not control or direct users' actions and are not responsible for the information or content shared, harm and/or action of the book readers.

Orange + Vanilla Soap

EOS
orange zest

CONTENTS

DISCLAIMER 3
CONTENTS 5
INTRODUCTION 1
BODY SCRUBS 5
    Benefits..5
    What you need 6
    Storage 7
    What to watch out for..7
BODY SCRUB RECIPES 9
    Your Go-To Basic Scrub 9
    Green Tea Scrub 10
    Chocolate Scrub 11
    Coffee Scrub..12
    Lemon Scrub 13
    Mint Chocolate Scrub 14
    Epsom Foot Scrub...15
    Rice and Honey Whitening Body Scrub 16
    Summer Red Lentil Body Scrub...............................17
    Red Lentil Body Scrub for winters...........................18
    Hydrating Body Scrub for Baby Soft Skin 19
    Face Whitening Scrub...20
    Lemon Lavender Body Scrub 21
    Anti-inflammatory Body Scrub 22

Scrub for Sensitive Skin 23

BODY LOTIONS..25

Benefits..26

Storage 26

How to do-it-yourself 27

What to watch out for...27

BODY LOTIONS RECIPES 29

Super Simple Luxurious Lotion 29

Lavender Lotion 31

Aloe Lotion..32

Double Chocolate Lotion 33

Raspberry Almond Lotion 35

Grapefruit Zing Lotion 37

Calamine Moisturiser 39

Baby Lotion 41

Sleep Time Lotion...43

Ultra Moisturizing Lotion..45

Organic Homemade Lotion Bar...47

Calendula Lotion 49

Nourishing Hand and Body Lotion 51

Ingredients 51

Nourishing Rose and Almond Moisturizer 52

BODY BUTTERS 53

Benefits..54

Storage 54

How to do-it-yourself 55

What to watch out for 55

BODY BUTTER RECIPES *57*

Hawaiian Body Butter 57

Mandarin Chocolate Body Butter 58

Strawberry Vanilla Butter..59

Golden Body Butter..61

Mango Body Butter 63

Cinnamon Body Butter 65

Citrus Body Butter for Glowing skin:......................................67

Vanilla Bean Body Butter..69

Anti-aging Face Cream..71

Aloe Vera Body Butter...73

Men after-shave cream 75

Stretch Mark lightening body butter 77

Rosemary Mint Whipped Shea Body Butter:..........................79

CONCLUSION *81*

MORE BOOKS FROM JOSEPHINE SIMON *83*

INTRODUCTION

The skin is the largest human organ of the human body, but it often doesn't get all the attention it deserves. It is time to change that because this very fact could be sucking some serious joy out of your life.

Here's why.

What's the first thing people see when they look at you? Your skin. Sure, other things like your beautiful eyes and pouty lips matter too, but not so much if they are surrounded by dry, crackly skin. No one wants to be "that guy/girl" that people avoid getting too close to for fear of accidentally touching sandpaper skin. Moreover, it feels good to have soft and luscious skin.

This is where a good skincare regime is necessary. You need to be nourishing your body from not only within, but also from the outside. A good skincare requires a variety of things including cleaning the skin to get rid of dead skin cells and hydrating the skin so that it remains supple and soft.

There are thousands of skincare products on the market. However, many of them contain harmful chemicals that might do the reverse of actually helping your skin. They may actually be hurting your skin. We have to remember that whatever it is that you place on your skin, seeps quickly into your body, so when you slather on a tube of something containing ingredients with long names you can't pronounce, you are probably absorbing chemicals into your body.

The absolute best way to ensure that you are getting clean, natural, wholesome ingredients in your skincare products are to go with all-natural, organic products. Store-bought products can cost you a pretty penny. However, there's another way. The amazingly simple, supremely cost-effective, and all-natural alternative to that is to make your beauty products at home.

That may sound daunting, but once you start doing it, you'll be amazed at how simple it truly is. You'll wonder why you didn't start concocting your own products a long time ago.

In this book, you will find directions and recipes for three very important components of your skincare regime: body scrubs, body lotions, and body butters. You need to exfoliate to get rid of dead skin cells to reveal the beautifully young and pliable ones underneath. This is where scrubs come in. The recipes included in this book will have you feeling refreshed, rejuvenated, and tingly all over with lovely concoctions like Mint Chocolate Scrub and our special Epsom Foot Scrub.

Retaining moisture in your skin is the ultimate necessity to younger looking skin, and that's where body lotions and body butters come in. These two help you to pull moisture from the air and get it into your skin as well as retain that moisture by creating a shield over the skin. We've combined the best of butters, oils, and essential oils to create all natural and balanced moisturizing for the skin with concoctions like Double Chocolate Lotion and Strawberry Vanilla Butter.

The fact of the matter is that the better the ingredients you put on your body, the better job your skin can do to protect you. This will be reflected in the way it glows, in its plumpness, and how soft it feels to the touch. This is the one thing you can easily do right away to help you look better, feel better, and walk with the confidence of a beautiful person on the inside and out.

BODY SCRUBS

The idea of exfoliating the skin so that it appears fresh and feels soft and supple can be traced back to one of the oldest medical documents in the world. The Ebers Papyrus is an ancient Egyptian scroll that details medical knowledge relating to everything from depression to how fluids are circulated in the body. It also sheds a light on the ancient Egyptian treatments for skin.

This is circa 1500 BC scroll also relays some of the Egyptian secrets for gorgeous skin including creating scrubs out of natural ingredients. Clearly, there is strong reason to believe that the simple concept of using some sort of abrasive natural materials to rid the skin of dead cells really does work and is an important part of any skincare regiment.

Benefits

Giving yourself a good scrub is akin to scraping off all the old, crusted bits from the bottom of a pot. Sure, at one time that skin that you're holding on to was fresh and new, but it's seen its heyday! When you slough it off, you're going to reveal a lovely new, soft layer underneath!

Getting rid of the old layer also means you're detoxifying the skin. In turn, your complexion glows. The sloughing off of the dead skin means fine lines disappear as the rough outer layer is eliminated. This elimination of the outer layer also has the added benefit of giving your skin a nice, clean appearance.

Cleaning the skin with a scrub also reduces oils and helps in preventing acne.

What you need

Scrubs are supremely easy to make at home! You need very few ingredients, which are probably already in your kitchen!

Exfoliant Ingredients
Sugar
Salt
Coffee grinds
Rice coarsely grinded
Nuts grinds

Lentil coarsely grinded

Moisturizing Ingredients

Extra virgin olive oil

Coconut oil

Coconut butter

Milk

Honey

Organic Ghee

Optional Ingredients

Essential oils (any that suits you)

Storage

Use an airtight jar to store your scrub. Generally Mason jars work great. You can package the scrub in small jars so you can avoid exposing your whole batch to the air each time you go to use one.

What to watch out for

Remember to do a small patch test on your skin before using the scrub all over your body to ensure you are not allergic to any of the ingredients.

BODY SCRUB RECIPES

Your Go-To Basic Scrub

This easy-to-recreate basic scrub includes ingredients you are likely to have in your kitchen. If you don't stock white sugar, you can substitute brown. Sugar is very beneficial when applied to the skin for a variety of reasons. One of the biggest is the AHA that it contains in abundance. This is the good stuff that is going to reduce those wrinkles and create a nice even tone!

Makes: 18 ounces

Ingredients
1½-cup organic cane sugar
¾ cup extra virgin olive oil *[handwritten: Grape Seed Oil]*
1 teaspoon vanilla extract

Directions
1. Combine ingredients in an airtight jar, mix well, and store in a cool place.
2. Moisten skin and scrub with mixture, wash off.

Green Tea ~~Green~~ Tree Scrub

Green tea oil provides numerous benefits to the skin. It has been used for everything from treating itching to a light form of UV protection. Its amazing antioxidant qualities make it an age-defying powerhouse. This green tea scrub provides just the right amount of anti-aging oil to green tea balance.

Makes: 18 ounces

Ingredients

1 ½ cup organic cane sugar
¾ cup coconut oil
1 tablespoon green tea essential oil
1 teaspoon tea tree oil

Directions

1. Combine ingredients in an airtight jar, mix well and store in a cool place.
2. Moisten skin and scrub with mixture, wash off.

Chocolate Scrub — For Angela

Cocoa not only smells divine, but it is also fantastic for the skin. Chocolate masks and baths have become popular due to cocoa's inherent antioxidant capabilities. When applied to the skin, these help to rid the body of skin-damaging free radicals.

Makes: 16 ounces

Ingredients

3 tablespoons organic cocoa powder
~~1 teaspoon cocoa essential~~ oil ✓
1¼-cup organic cane sugar
¾ cup coconut oil

Directions

1. Combine ingredients in an airtight jar, mix well, and store in a cool place.
2. Moisten skin and scrub with mixture, wash off.

Coffee Scrub

Now you can have your coffee and drink it too with this wonderfully aromatic coffee scrub made out of coffee grounds! The coffee grounds stimulate the skin. It's also believed that rubbing the grounds on cellulite helps to reduce it!

Makes: 12 ounces

Ingredients

½ cup coffee grounds
1 cup coconut oil / almond oil / palm oil
1 teaspoon vanilla extract

cinnamon

Directions

1. Combine ingredients in an airtight jar, mix well and store in a cool place.
2. Moisten skin and scrub with mixture, wash off.

Lemon Scrub

Drop a little lemon into your scrub, and you'll see it do amazing things for your skin – like magic. Rub the lemony scrub onto your elbows and knees and watch the dark spots disappear! Additionally, lemon's astringent properties help to truly clean the skin and make it brighter.

Makes: 12 ounces

chopped.
+ lemon balm

Ingredients

2 teaspoons lemon peel, grated

1 tablespoon lemon juice

1 cup organic cane sugar

2 teaspoons vitamin E

½ cup coconut oil

Directions

1. Combine ingredients in an airtight jar, mix well, and store in a cool place.
2. Moisten skin and scrub with mixture, wash off.

Scrub this on your body in the morning, and be prepared to have the wheels in your head turning at ultimate speeds all day! The scent of peppermint has a big, positive affect on mental function in ways such as improving memory and focus.

Makes: 12 ounces

Ingredients
1-cup organic cane sugar
½ cup almond oil
2 tablespoons pure cocoa powder
1 teaspoon peppermint essential oil

Directions
1. Combine ingredients in an airtight jar, mix well and store in a cool place.
2. Moisten skin and scrub with mixture, wash off.

Epsom Foot Scrub

Dry, hardened spots on the skin are terrible to touch and pretty horrible to look at. They can be disheartening personally and quite embarrassing. This is why you must absolutely use this scrub to make your feet beautiful and lovely. Epsom salt is anti-fungal and helps to deodorize feet. In addition, the minerals also help to alleviate pain and discomfort. Your feet work hard for you so it is definitely time to show them some love.

Makes: 12 ounces

Ingredients
¾ cup Epsom salt
¼ cup sea salt
½ cup coconut oil

Directions
1. Combine ingredients in an airtight jar, mix well and store in a cool place.
2. Moisten skin and scrub with mixture, wash off

...e and Honey Whitening Body Scrub

Rice powder has excellent exfoliating properties; it also helps in brightening skin tone. Honey is one of the best organic products for your skin. It works as an anti-bacterial and anti-aging product. It opens up the pores and it is a good natural moisturizer that soothes your skin. It makes your skin glow and makes it soft and supple to touch.

Makes: 12 ounces

Ingredients
1 cup rice, ground coarsely
3 tablespoons honey
10-12 drops almond oil (use only for dry skin)

Directions
1. Combine ingredients in an airtight jar, mix well and store in a cool place.
2. Moisten skin and scrub with mixture for a couple of minutes, then wash off.

Summer Red Lentil Body Scrub

Rose water helps you feel refreshed during summertime. It provides relief for itchiness or a burning sensation. Honey is a good moisturizer, an anti-oxidant, and an antibacterial too. It suits all types of skin and makes your skin supple. The red lentils help remove dead skin cells from your skin and also give to add a healthy glow.

Makes: 12 ounces

Ingredients
½ cup red lentils, ground coarsely
3 tablespoons honey
2 tablespoons rose water

Directions

1. Combine ingredients in an airtight jar, mix well and store in a cool place.
2. Moisten skin and scrub with mixture, wash off.

Red Lentil Body Scrub for winters

Winters can rob your skin of its natural moisture. If you have dry skin, then moisturising won't be enough. That is where using organic ghee comes to the rescue, Organic Ghee is considered as a natural skin moisturiser. It works wonders on dry skin, making it soft and supple. The red lentils help remove dead skin cells from your skin and also give to add a healthy glow.

Makes: 12 ounces

Ingredients
1 cup red lentils, ground coarsely
½ cup ghee
Rose essential oil (since ghee can have a strong aroma)

Directions

1. Combine ingredients in an airtight jar, mix well and store in a cool place.
2. Moisten skin and scrub with mixture, wash off.

Hydrating Body Scrub for Baby Soft Skin

This body scrub is full of goodness. Aloe Vera works wonders for moisturizing your skin, it works very well on dry skin in particular. It is a good skin conditioner and is rich in vitamin E. It nourishes your skin and helps prevent wrinkles. Walnuts are loaded with vitamins and minerals that are great for the skin. Almonds are good source of vitamin E. It prevents wrinkles and gives a healthy glow to your skin. Honey is a great moisturiser for all types of skin.

Makes: 6 ounces.

Preparation time: 5 minutes

Ingredients
1 leaf of aloe vera
~~A handful of walnuts~~
A handful of almonds
2 tablespoons honey

Directions
1. Remove the pulp from the aloe vera leaf
2. Grind together all the ingredients to get a coarse paste.
3. Apply the mixture on the skin. Leave it on for 5 minutes. Scrub lightly in circular motions.
4. Wash off with lukewarm water.
5. Always make the scrub fresh and use. Discard leftovers. Use it once a week for a soft and supple skin

Face Whitening Scrub

Milk is a natural skin moisturiser; it especially works well on dry skin. People with oily skin should avoid this scrub, as it will make your face oilier. Rice powder helps in getting rid of dead skin cells and also known to whiten your skin tone.

Makes: 12 ounces

Ingredients
½ cup rice, powdered coarsely
½ cup lukewarm milk

Directions
1. Mix the rice powder and milk together in a bowl to form a paste.
2. Apply on the face and scrub in circular motion, best to use this scrub at night.
3. Wash off with lukewarm water, your face may feel a bit oily for the time being, but the 'natural oils' from the milk will be soaked in a skin and you will be left with a fresh and dewy face the next morning.

Lemon Lavender Body Scrub

Scrubs are not just for getting rid of dead skin cells. Body scrubs are known to help relieve tension and let the body relax. Epsom salt used in the scrub relaxes your muscles and also helps reduce inflammation. Olive oil keeps the skin moist. Lemon juice acts as a bleaching agent, while the Lavender helps you relax your senses. This is a relaxing body scrub and helps relieve the tension from your body. A perfect scrub that works on your body and also lets your mind relax.

Makes: 12 ounces.

Ingredients
1 ¼ cup Epsom salt or coarse salt crystals
¼ cup ~~olive oil~~ *grape seed oil*
¼ cup lemon juice
1 tablespoon lavender essential oil

Directions
1. Combine ingredients in an airtight jar, mix well and store in a cool place.
2. Moisten skin and scrub with mixture, wash off.

4 jars

Anti-inflammatory Body Scrub

Turmeric has anti-inflammatory and anti-bacterial properties that soothes your skin and helps fight skin bacteria. Essential oils (depending on the type you choose) have their own skin care and relaxation benefits. Sugar and salt will help get rid of the dead skin cells.

Makes: 25 ounces.

Ingredients:
1 ½ cups salt
1 ½ cups sugar
3 tablespoons turmeric powder
6-8 drops essential oil of your choice

Directions

1. Combine ingredients in an airtight jar, mix well and store in a cool place.
2. Moisten skin and scrub with mixture, wash off.

Scrub for Sensitive Skin

Avocado is rich in natural oils that help moisturise skin. Cucumber is known for its oil removal properties and is also a natural coolant. It has skin whitening properties. It also gives relief to skin burns and other skin inflammations. Brown sugar is an excellent dead skin cell remover.

Makes: 12 ounces.

Ingredients
1 cup brown sugar
½ cup avocado oil
1 medium cucumber, chopped into pieces

Directions
1. Blend the cucumber pieces in a blender until smooth.
2. Mix together in a bowl, the blended cucumber, avocado oil and brown sugar
3. Rub it gently all over your body. Leave it on for 3-4 minutes.
4. Wash with lukewarm water.

BODY LOTIONS

All market lotions are not created equal! Creating your own at home is absolutely the best option.

Lotions are designed to moisturize the skin, but some store-bought brands can actually leave the skin drier than it was before. This can happen when the lotion is made up of inexpensive materials that do not, in fact, lock the moisture in. These lotions dissipate quickly, leaving your skin drier than before.

Body Lotions are made up of three components. The first, the humectant component, sucks water from the air and into your skin. The second, the occlusive component, helps to seal in that moisture. The third component is designed to help your skin replenish itself.

Body lotions provide moisture for the skin and help to prevent cracking and chapping. Lotions are in the same family as creams, however, they're not quite as viscose. This low-viscosity factor means you can use them all over the body for total moisturizing. Lotions can also be easily applied after hand washing and will help them stay smooth, soft, and appear youthful.

Benefits

Body lotions are a great option for full-body moisturizing.

The lotions you will be making at home contain essential ingredients that hone in on what your skin needs and then replenish what's missing. Since you will be using only the best of ingredients, these high-quality lotions also seal your skin so you aren't losing any moisturizer either.

The combination of the moisturizer with essential oils that are mood stabilizers and contain other properties to promote skin health make for a fantastic skincare product you can count on.

Storage

If possible, try to get yourself a pump bottle so you avoid contamination. However, if you can't find one, you can use jars with airtight lids.

How to do-it-yourself

Creating body lotion at home is a snap, you need a few simple ingredients, a blender, and soon you'll have gorgeous body lotion at a fraction of the cost of over-the-counter brands.

You will use a combination of the following ingredients:

Distilled water
Aloe Vera
Oil
Beeswax
Essential oil

What to watch out for

Since we are trying to make these body lotions as clean and good for you as possible, we haven't included any of the chemicals that commercial brands use. However, that also means the lotions are more vulnerable to contamination. In order to prevent contamination, it is best to use the pump-bottle option. You should be able to easily find them on the web. If you do end up using a jar, make sure your hands are clean each time you use the product in order to minimize the chance of contamination. Also make sure you dry your hands after washing them in order to avoid contaminating the lotion with water bacteria.

BODY LOTIONS RECIPES

Super Simple Luxurious Lotion

This particular lotion is a little heavier than your standard one, so you will need to place the lotion in a container as opposed to a pump bottle. The grape seed oil extract is a natural preservative, meaning you can store this lotion for a lot longer than you would most homemade products.

Makes: 16 ounces

Ingredients
1 cup ~~almond~~ oil PALM OIL
½ cup coconut oil
½ cup beeswax
1 teaspoon vanilla extract
½ teaspoon grape seed oil extract

Directions
1. Place ingredients in a clean glass jar.
2. Create a water bath in a saucepan, and place jar in saucepan, allow ingredients to melt.
3. Mix ingredients and place in your sterilized containers.

4. You can store this lotion unopened for approximately 24 week.

Lavender Lotion

There's something about lavender that makes it a wonderfully soothing scent. Lavender in essential oil form is believed to help in mild cases of depression. Additionally, the topical application of it has healing qualities and is antiseptic.

Makes: 16 ounces

Ingredients

1-cup coconut oil

1 cup Shea butter

2 teaspoons lavender essential oil

Directions

1. Place ingredients in a clean glass jar.
2. Create a water bath in a saucepan and place the jar in the saucepan and allow ingredients to melt.
3. Mix ingredients and place in your sterilized containers.

Aloe Lotion

Aloe is wonderfully soothing for irritated skin is found in numerous commercial applications. The great news is that you can enjoy the healing benefits of aloe without the additional gunk that commercial products have by mixing up your very own batch.

Makes: 14 ounces
Preparation time: 5 minutes

Ingredients
¼ cup pure Aloe Vera gel
1 cup coconut oil
½ cup grated beeswax
1 teaspoon Vitamin E oil

Directions
1. Place ingredients in saucepan and heat over low heat.
2. As ingredients melt, mix.
3. Once ingredients are melted, remove pot to counter, and rest for 10 minutes.
4. Place lotion for immediate use in dispenser and remainder in a jar with an airtight lid.

Double Chocolate Lotion

The scent of this lotion is absolutely divine. Get yourself a tiny bottle and fill it up with lotion so you can carry it with you and apply after washing your hands. This simple thing can help in slowing down the aging look of hands.

Makes: 14 ounces
Preparation time: 5 minutes

Ingredients

1 teaspoon cocoa essential oil
½ cup pure distilled water
½ cup cocoa butter
½ cup jojoba oil
½ cup grated beeswax
1 teaspoon Vitamin E oil

Directions

1. Place ingredients in saucepan and heat over low heat.
2. As ingredients melt, mix.
3. Once ingredients are melted, remove pot to counter and rest for 10 minutes.

4. Place lotion for immediate use in dispenser and remainder in a jar with an airtight lid.

Raspberry Almond Lotion

Raspberry seed oil is a powerhouse of antioxidants and includes the wonderfully beneficial Omega-3 and Omega-6 oils. Make sure that you are buying raspberry seed oil and not raspberry oil. There is no such natural product in existence, so you will be slathering your body with synthetic raspberry.

Makes: 14 ounces
Preparation time: 5 minutes

Ingredients

2 teaspoons raspberry seed oil
¼ cup pure Aloe Vera gel
1 cup almond oil
½ cup grated beeswax
1 teaspoon vitamin E oil

Directions

1. Place ingredients in saucepan and heat over low heat.
2. As ingredients melt, stir continuously until well mixed.
3. Once ingredients are melted, remove pot to counter and rest for 10 minutes.

4. Place lotion for immediate use in dispenser and remainder in a jar with an airtight lid.

Grapefruit Zing Lotion

Say "Good morning!" to yourself with the refreshing scent of grapefruit. This scent not only packs a punch, but the essential oil helps you avoid getting those aesthetically worrying pimples.

Makes: 14 ounces
Preparation time: 5 minutes

Ingredients

1 teaspoon grapefruit essential oil
¼ cup pure Aloe Vera Gel
1-cup coconut oil
½ cup grated beeswax
1 teaspoon Vitamin E oil

Directions

1. Place ingredients in saucepan and heat over low heat.
2. As ingredients melt, mix.
3. Once ingredients are melted, remove pot to counter and rest for 10 minutes.
4. Place lotion for immediate use in dispenser and remainder in a jar with an airtight lid.

Calamine Moisturiser

Calamine lotion is a multipurpose lotion, which can be used for sunburns; insect bites, dressing wounds etc. Bentonite clay helps in healing wounds faster. Baking soda helps relieve itching and skin irritation. Tea tree oil soothes inflamed or itchy skin. Sea salt helps reduce swelling and removes dead skin cells. Pink kaolin clay is helpful for sensitive skin. It is an excellent exfoliator. It gives color to the lotion. Glycerine helps absorb moisture into the skin.

Makes: 12 ounces

Preparation time: 5 minutes

Ingredients:

1 cup water or more if required

16 teaspoons bentonite clay

16 teaspoons baking soda

4 tablespoons sea salt

40 drops tea tree essential oil

4 teaspoons glycerine (optional)

10 teaspoons kaolin clay

Directions

1. Mix together baking soda, salt, bentonite clay and kaolin in a bowl.
2. Add water and stir constantly so as to form a paste.
3. Add more water if required until the desired consistency is achieved.
4. Add tea tree oil and glycerine and mix well.
5. Store in an airtight jar in a cool and dry place.

Baby Lotion

Coconut oil is a great natural moisturiser, which helps fight wrinkles and deep nourishes your skin. Aloe Vera has anti-inflammatory and moisturising properties. Olive oil and vitamin E oil works wonders for a soft and supple and younger looking skin. Lanolin helps cure skin abrasions and also deep moisturises your skin.

Makes: 16 ounces.

Ingredients

1 cup water

¼ cup olive oil

2 tablespoons coconut oil

2 tablespoons beeswax, grated

1 vitamin E capsule

1 tablespoon shea butter or cocoa butter

½ teaspoon Aloe Vera

½ teaspoon 100% lanolin

Directions

1. Place ingredients in a clean glass jar.

2. Create a water bath in a saucepan and place a jar in it and allow the ingredients to melt.
3. Mix all the ingredients and place in your sterilized containers.

Sleep Time Lotion

This lotion is very helpful for people with insomnia. Chamomile is an anti-inflammatory and has anti-bacterial properties. It helps heal rough and damaged skin. It has properties that help you soothe your mind and relaxes your senses. The soothing smell of lavender helps to relax, sleep faster and reduce stress. Jojoba oil helps to keep the skin softer.

Makes: 12 ounces.

Preparation time: 3 hours

Ingredients

1 ½ ounce coconut oil

3 ounces liquid jojoba oil, infused

¾ ounce bees wax, grated

2 ½ teaspoons chamomile flowers

2 ½ teaspoons lavender buds

4 ounces distilled water, heated

10 drops chamomile essential oil

10 drops lavender essential oil

Cheesecloth

Directions

1. To infuse the oil, place chamomile flowers and lavender buds in a clean jar like a Mason jar. Pour jojoba oil on top. Place the lid and tightly close it.
2. Create a water bath in a saucepan and place the jar in the simmering water. Let it sit in the simmering water bath for about 2 hours. Remove from heat and let it cool down. Strain the infused oil through a cheesecloth. Discard the flowers and the buds.
3. Pour hot water in a tall container. Place a stick blender in the container on low speed.
4. With the blender running slowly, pour the infused oil in a thin drizzle into the container.
5. It will slowly start getting creamy.
6. Now add the essential oils. Stop the blender when you reach the consistency you desire.
7. Spoon it into an airtight container. Store in a cool and dry place.

Ultra Moisturizing Lotion

Shea butter is well known for its skin moisturising properties. It helps reduce wrinkles and also treats eczema and other such skin conditions. Tea tree oil is an anti-bacterial that helps fight pimples and maintain a blemish free skin. The essential oils help soothe the skin and also relax the senses. Almond oil is rich in vitamin E, which can very well be called an elixir for younger looking skin.

Makes: 12 ounces

Ingredients

1 cup Shea butter

4 tablespoons avocado oil or sweet almond oil or jojoba oil

30 drops lavender essential oil

20 drops rosemary essential oil

15 drops carrot seed oil

10 drops tea tree oil

Directions

1. Place a saucepan over medium low heat. Add Shea butter and the essential oil of your choice. When it is melted, remove from heat. Transfer into a bowl.
2. Place the bowl in the freezer to cool for about 15-20 minutes until it is slightly solid.
3. Add lavender oil, rosemary oil, carrot seed oil, and tea tree oil. Whisk until the mixture is creamy. (You can use the whisk attachment of your mixer or you can use a hand whisk)
4. Spoon into a clean and dry jar. Store it in a cool and dry place at room temperature.
5. Apply on the body as well as face whenever required.

Organic Homemade Lotion Bar

Coconut oil is known for its skin nourishing and wrinkle fighting abilities. Shea butter is a natural moisturiser that is one of the best natural skin care ingredients. Vitamin E helps rebuild skin cells and keeps your skin soft, supple and younger. Beeswax helps fights acne and also skin conditions like eczema and psoriasis.

Makes: 24 ounces.
Preparation time: 5 minutes

Ingredients

8 ounces coconut oil

8 ounces Shea butter or cocoa butter or mango butter or a mixture of all the 3 butters

8 ounces beeswax or more if you like a thicker consistency

3 teaspoons vitamin E oil

10-15 drops essential oil of your choice

Directions

1. Mix all the ingredients except essential oil and vitamin E oil in a heat resistant glass bowl.

2. Boil some water in a saucepan and place the bowl on top when the water is simmering. Allow ingredients to melt.
3. Add essential oil and vitamin E oil.
4. Mix ingredients gently with your hands and pour into moulds of desired shape.
5. Let it cool completely before removing it out of the mould. These bars are ideal for gifting.

Calendula Lotion

Calendula helps heal wounds and cuts faster. Beeswax actively fights acne and pimple causing bacteria. It is a natural skin moisturiser that keeps your skin soft and supple. Glycerine is one of the best natural ingredients to moisturise your skin. Grape seed oil has anti-wrinkle properties.

Makes: 18 ounces

Ingredients

8 ounces jojoba oil, calendula infused

8 ounces distilled water, calendula infused

1 ounce beeswax

1 ounce glycerine

1 ounce witch hazel

½ teaspoon grapefruit seed extract (optional)

20 drops lavender essential oil (optional)

10 drops rosemary essential oil

5-6 handfuls Calendula flowers fresh or dried about 5-6 teaspoons

Directions

1. To infuse the oil: place half the calendula flowers in a clean jar, like a Mason jar. Pour jojoba oil over it. Place the lid and tightly close it.
2. Create a water bath in a saucepan and place the jar in the saucepan. Let it remain in the water bath simmering for about 2 hours.
3. Once it is infused, strain it through a cheesecloth. Discard the flowers.
4. Meanwhile, prepare the calendula infused water as follows: Place the remaining calendula flowers in a bowl. Pour boiling hot distilled water over it. Allow it to steep. When it attains room temperature, strain and use the water. Discard the flowers.
5. To a heat resistant bowl, add witch hazel, infused jojoba oil, beeswax and glycerine. Place the bowl over a water bath.
6. Allow the ingredients to melt. Mix thoroughly.
7. Remove the bowl from the water bath.
8. Add the infused water. With an immersion blender set on low, start mixing.
9. It will start getting creamy. Add rosemary oil, lavender oil and grapefruit seed extract. Stop the blender when you reach the consistency you desire. Transfer into an airtight jar.

Nourishing Hand and Body Lotion

Shea Butter and coconut oil are excellent natural skin moisturisers that help you maintain soft and supple skin. Coconut oil deep nourishes skin. Aloe Vera helps fight skin inflammation and has anti-bacterial properties.

Makes: 12 ounces.

Ingredients

½ cup coconut oil

¼ cup Shea butter

¼ cup cocoa butter

2 tablespoons aloe Vera juice

2 tablespoons jojoba oil

10 drops essential oil of your choice

Directions

1. Add Shea butter, coconut oil, and coconut butter to a saucepan. Place the saucepan over low heat. When the ingredients have melted, remove from heat.
2. Add aloe Vera, jojoba oil, and essential oil. Whisk well until you get the desired consistency.
3. Transfer into an airti
4. ght container and store in a cool dry place.

Nourishing Rose and Almond Moisturizer

Shea Butter, cocoa butter and coconut oil are excellent natural skin moisturisers that help you maintain soft and supple skin. Almond oil helps nourish the skin from within and has reduces fine lines and wrinkles.

Makes: 12 ounces.

Ingredients

½ cup coconut oil
¼ cup Shea butter
¼ cup cocoa butter
2 tablespoons rose water
2 tablespoons almond oil
10 drops rose essential oil

Directions

1. Add Shea butter, coconut oil, and coconut butter to a saucepan. Place the pan over low heat. When the ingredients are melted, remove from heat.
2. Add rose, almond oil, and rose essential oil. Whisk well until you get the desired consistency.
3. Transfer into an airtight container and store in a cool dry place.

BODY BUTTERS

Body butter is intended to be as decadent as it sounds. It provides your skin with a full blast of moisture thanks to the high oil content. Body butters differ from lotions in that they are much thicker and are able to provide your skin with a thicker barrier against moisture loss. Body butters have been known since Roman times. Those body butters are similar in composition to the recipes provided in this book in that the ingredients are all natural without the harmful preservatives found in commercial products.

We've used a variety of butters including Shea butter, mango butter, and coconut butter as the base for our body butter recipes. These butters contain essential vitamins and antioxidants that are not only replenishing but also healing. The high viscosity levels make the butters quite dense and perfect for very dry areas. It is also a good idea to give your whole body the body butter treatment once a week to get amazingly soft, supple skin all over.

Benefits

Body butters provide ultimate moisturizing for ultimate beauty. They are composed of humectants and occlusive agents like body lotions but the composition in butters comes in at a ratio that really takes their effect on the skin right off the charts.

Common humectants found in body butter include honey and glycerine. These do the heavy lifting when it comes to luring moisture from the air into your skin.

Common occlusives include Shea butter and silicone. The occlusives are your official skin guards, which ensure that once the moisture has made its way into your skin, it stays there.

Storage

Use mason jars or another type of jar with an airtight lid to store your body butters. You should sterilize the waters in a water bath prior to filling and sealing them. Once sealed, store them in a cool place.

How to do-it-yourself

Body butters are simple to make at home and require little time.

Standard body butters include a combination of the following elements:

Butter

Oil

Essential oil

What to watch out for

The thick consistency of body butter means you need to use jars for storage, and of course, that means that contamination is possible. It is best to store your butter in smaller jars so that the chance of contamination per jar is less. Also ensure that you have clean, dry hands before you stick your hand into one of the jars to scoop out some body butter.

BODY BUTTER RECIPES

Hawaiian Body Butter

Slather summer on your body with this body butter scented by pineapple and mango. The mango butter is wonderfully rich. Its anti-aging properties can reduce those irritating lines that begin to appear as you age. The mango butter combined with coconut oil and Vitamin E will have you feeling lovely and soft.

Serves: 12 ounces

Ingredients

1 teaspoon pineapple essential oil
½ cup mango butter
1 cup coconut oil
1 teaspoon vitamin E oil

Directions

1. Place ingredients in a glass bowl and beat until smooth.
2. Scoop butter into sterilized jars and store in a cool place.

Mandarin Chocolate Body Butter

Raise your hands if you absolutely love the heavenly scent of mandarin spiked with chocolate! This body butter is fantastic on the skin. The natural scents provide a mood boost that will have you whipping through the morning and afternoon in sweet haze.

Makes: 12 ounces

Ingredients

1 teaspoon mandarin zest

1 teaspoon cocoa essential oil

1 ½ cups coconut butter

Directions

1. Place ingredients in a glass bowl and beat until smooth.
2. Scoop butter into sterilized jars and store in a cool place.

Strawberry Vanilla Butter

Stay sweet all day long with lovely strawberry and vanilla-infused butter. Strawberries contain ellagic acid that helps spur the production of collagen and in turn ensures you age more slowly. As in the case of raspberry seed essential oil, there is no such thing as strawberry essential oil, you must be sure to purchase only strawberry seed essential oil to ensure you're getting an all-natural product.

Makes: 16 ounces

Ingredients

2 teaspoons strawberry seed essential oil
1 cup Shea butter
½ cup coconut oil
½ cup jojoba oil

Directions

1. Fill a saucepan halfway up with water and heat over medium.
2. Grab a glass bowl that will fit over the mouth of the saucepan.
3. Place Shea butter and coconut oil in glass bowl, stir until melted.

4. Remove bowl and place on cool surface.
5. Add oils, stir, and cool in refrigerator for half an hour.
6. Once mixture is cool, use a hand immersion blender to beat butter until cream.
7. Scoop butter into jars with airtight lids and store in a cool place until use.

Golden Body Butter

Oh how she glows and she glows. You will glow after using this butter thanks to the cocoa powder and honey combination, which creates a slightly sun-kissed look.

Makes: 16 ounces

Ingredients

2 tablespoons cocoa powder

2 tablespoons raw honey

1 cup Shea butter

½ cup coconut oil

½ cup jojoba oil

Directions

1. Fill a saucepan halfway up with water and heat over medium.
2. Grab a glass bowl that will fit over the mouth of the saucepan.
3. Place Shea butter and coconut oil in glass bowl, stir until melted.
4. Remove bowl and place on cool surface.
5. Add remaining ingredients, stir, and cool in refrigerator for half an hour.

6. Once mixture is cool, use a hand immersion blender to beat butter until cream.
7. Scoop butter into jars with airtight lids and store in a cool place until use.

Mango Body Butter

This simple, rich butter is great to use in the winter. After taking a shower, slather it all over your feet, don your socks, and wake up in the morning with feet so soft you'll feel as though you can float!

Makes: 14 ounces

Ingredients

1 cup mango butter
½ cup coconut oil
1 teaspoon vitamin E oil
2 tablespoons aloe gel

Directions

1. Fill a saucepan halfway up with water and heat over medium.
2. Grab a glass bowl that will fit over the mouth of the saucepan.
3. Place mango butter and coconut oil in glass bowl, stir until it melts.
4. Remove bowl and place on cool surface.
5. Add remaining ingredients, stir, and cool in refrigerator for half an hour.

6. Once mixture is cool, use a hand immersion blender to beat butter until cream.
7. Scoop butter into jars with airtight lids and store in a cool place until use.

Cinnamon Body Butter

The comfy scent of cinnamon can make you feel at home wherever you are. When used in a lotion, it will give you that same feeling of cozy comfort. Cinnamon is also wonderful for the skin with anti-bacterial properties. It's great for soothing skin as well as soothing joints.

Makes: 12 ounces

Ingredients

1 teaspoon cinnamon essential oil
1 teaspoon Arabica seed oil
1 cup cocoa butter
½ cup Argan oil

Directions

1. Fill a saucepan halfway up with water and heat over medium.
2. Grab a glass bowl that will fit over the mouth of the saucepan.
3. Place cocoa butter and coconut oil in glass bowl, stir until melted.
4. Remove bowl and place on cool surface.
5. Add remaining ingredients, stir, and cool in refrigerator for half an hour.

6. Once mixture is cool, use a hand immersion blender to beat butter until cream.
7. Scoop butter into jars with airtight lids and store in a cool place until use.

Citrus Body Butter for Glowing skin:

Tea tree oil is an anti-bacterial. The extra virgin coconut oil and Shea butter will provide your skin with the moisture it needs throughout the day. The orange essential oil will keep your mind fresh and alert.

Makes: 35 ounces.

Ingredients

3 cups extra virgin coconut Oil

10.5 ounces Shea Butter

5 drops tea tree oil

20 drops sweet orange essential oil

20 drops lemon essential oil

Directions

1. Mix Shea butter and coconut oil in a jar like a Mason jar. Cover tightly the jar with lid.
2. Create a water bath in a saucepan and place the jar in the saucepan. Allow all the ingredients to melt.

3. Remove from heat and add the tea tree oil and essential oils. Mix well and cool for about 30 minutes.
4. Freeze the mixture for 10-15 minutes or more. When the oils slightly start solidifying, remove from freezer and whip with a whisk until you get a light buttery consistency.
5. Spoon into a clean jar. Close the lid tightly and place in a cool dry area.

Vanilla Bean Body Butter

This body butter will make you feel rejuvenated throughout the day, thanks to the pleasant and soothing aroma of vanilla. It also helps relax the body and mind. The cocoa butter helps to deep nourish the skin and the almond oil provides it with the much needed Vitamin E oil.

Makes: 16 ounces.

Ingredients

1 cup raw cocoa butter

½ cup sweet almond oil

½ cup coconut oil

2 vanilla bean pods

Directions

1. Add cocoa butter and coconut oil to a pan. Place the pan over low heat. When the ingredients are melted, remove from heat and keep aside to cool.
2. Grind the vanilla bean in a coffee grinder or food processor.
3. Add sweet almond oil and ground vanilla beans to the cooled cocoa butter coconut oil mixture. Mix well and freeze for about 20-25 minutes.

4. Whip in a food processor until buttery and creamy.
5. Scoop into a glass jar with a lid. Refrigerate and use when necessary.

Anti-aging Face Cream

Shea butter restores the skin moisture. Rose water rejuvenates the skin. Honey and beeswax will retain the moisture and also help fight signs of aging. Wheat germ tightens skin cells and improves it elasticity.

Makes: 7-8 ounces.

Ingredients

8 teaspoons beeswax, grated

4 tablespoons rosewater

~~¼ cup shea butter~~ — palm oil

8 teaspoons wheat germ oil

4 tablespoons sweet almond oil

~~4 teaspoons organic honey~~ Honey?

10 drops carrot seed oil

10 drops rose oil, or any essential oil of your choice

Handwritten notes: x5 = 500, %10, 20mL, 76 hrs, ¼ cup 50 mL, palm oil 20mL, Honey?

Directions

1. Place the beeswax in a glass container. Place the container on a double boiler on low heat.
2. Pour the rosewater in a cup and place the cup in the double boiler along with the beeswax. Similarly warm the honey.

3. When beeswax is melted, add shea butter and stir constantly until it melts and is well blended.
4. Add wheat germ oil and sweet almond oil. Whip with an immersion blender or hand mixer until the mixture is well blended. Add the warmed rose water and honey slowly, whipping simultaneously.
5. Remove from the heat. Stir constantly until it is cooled.
6. Add essential oils. Stir well.
7. Scoop it into a glass jar. Cover tightly with a lid.

Aloe Vera Body Butter

Aloe Vera soothes the skin and prevents skin inflammation. The 3 butters will provide your skin with the much-needed moisture and will keep your skin soft and supple. The essential oils will relax your mind and body. The grapeseed oil and beeswax will help prevent skin conditions like rashes, eczema and acne.

Makes: 30 ounces.

Ingredients

6 ounces shea butter

4 ounces mango butter

2 ounces coconut butter

2 ounces coconut oil

6 ounces grapeseed oil

1 ounce beeswax

4 ounces distilled water

4 ounces aloe Vera gel

40 drops sweet orange essential oil

40 drops patchouli essential oil

20 drops lavender essential oil

Directions

1. Mix the Shea butter, mango butter, coconut butter, coconut oil, grapeseed oil and beeswax in a heat resistant glass bowl.
2. Create a water bath in a saucepan and place the bowl over the saucepan. Allow all the ingredients to melt.
3. Remove the mixture from heat and let it cool for a while.
4. Place an immersion blender or hand mixer in the bowl. Let it run on low speed.
5. Slowly pour the water and aloe Vera gel. The mixture will become homogenous and creamy once you start blending. Continue blending until it mixes well.
6. Add in the essential oils. Mix well until you reach the desired consistency.
7. Spoon into sterilized jars. Close the lid tightly and store in a cool and dry place.

Men after-shave cream

This one is specifically for the men out there, as it makes an excellent after-shave cream. It helps to soothe irritated and inflamed skin. Tea tree oil has anti-fungal and anti-bacterial properties. The coconut oil and Shea butter will deep nourish your skin.

Makes: 30 ounces.

Ingredients

1 ½ cups coconut oil

18 tablespoons cocoa butter [handwritten: Palm oil]

6 tablespoons jojoba oil

40 drops tea tree oil

50 drops lavender essential oil or any essential oil of your choice

Directions

1. Add the cocoa butter to a bowl. Place the bowl over a saucepan with simmering water. When it is melted, remove it from heat.
2. Add coconut oil, jojoba oil and lavender essential oil. Stir well.
3. Place the mixture in the refrigerator for a while.

4. When the oil mixture slightly begins to solidify, whip with a whisk until you get a buttery and creamy consistency. You can also put it in a blender and blend on high speed pulsing every 10 seconds until the mixture becomes light and fluffy.
5. Add tea tree oil once you are done with the whipping.
6. Spoon it into a glass jar. Cover the mixture with a tight lid.
7. Store in a cool and dry place.

Stretch Mark lightening body butter

Regular use of this butter helps to lighten stretch marks.

Makes: 22 ounces

Ingredients

1 cup cocoa butter

1 cup shea butter

6 tablespoons almond oil

6 tablespoons olive oil

20 drops of lavender essential oil

20 drops of geranium essential oil

20 drops of patchouli essential oil

Directions

1. Add Shea butter and cocoa butter to a heat resistant glass bowl.
2. Prepare a water bath in a saucepan. Place bowl over the saucepan when the water is simmering. Let the butters melt.

3. When completely melted, slowly add almond oil and olive oil. Stir well. Remove from heat and cool for about ½ an hour.
4. Add essential oils. Stir well.
5. Place the mixture in the freezer for a while.
6. When the oils slightly begin to solidify, whip with a whisk or an immersion blender until you get a buttery consistency.
7. Scoop it into a glass jar. Cover tightly with a lid.
8. Store in a cool and dry place.

Rosemary Mint Whipped Shea Body Butter:

This body butter provides long lasting moisture. It is ideal for dry and chapped skin. The kukui nut oil, extracted from the Hawaiian native tree Aleurites moluccans, also known as the candlenut tree, helps soothing and softening the skin and relief from eczema and psoriasis skin conditions as well as sunburns. The spearmint and rosemary oil will sharpen your senses and keep you feeling fresh all day long.

Makes: 30 ounces.

Ingredients

6 ounces cocoa butter

18 ounces shea butter

6 ounces kukui nut oil

50 drops spearmint essential oil

40 drops rosemary essential oil

Directions

1. In a heat resistant glass bowl, place the cocoa butter. Add Shea butter and kukui nut oil.
2. Place the bowl over a water bath over low heat.
3. When the butters are melted, remove from heat. Keep aside to cool at room temperature.

4. Place it in the freezer for about 20 minutes until it almost solidify.
5. Whisk the mixture with a metal whisk or an immersion blender on low speed.
6. Freeze it again for 15-20 minutes.
7. The color will start getting creamy.
8. Whisk again and place it in the freezer if necessary until the mixture is absolutely chilled and has reached the desired consistency.
9. Add the essential oils. Mix well.
10. Spoon it into glass jars.
11. Keep in a cool and dark place.

CONCLUSION

You get one body in this lifetime and that body is covered with one of your hardest-working organs, your skin! Your skin is a shield from the elements and regulates what your body takes in from the environment. Much of the pollution in the air consists of particles that we can't see but that our skin filters for us. With your skin doing all of this heavy lifting, it is absolutely essential you give it the right food to function and maintain.

Body scrubs help get rid of skin that is dead and in turn reveal the plump, soft, baby skin underneath. Lotions and butters help to pull moisture in, which is absolutely essential for youthful, glowing skin. Butters help to create a nice, thick, protective layer to retain moisture that is going to ensure your shield, aka your skin, is in top form.

The ease of creating skincare products at home will make you an absolute believer that homemade is best. Beyond the ease is that fact that the recipes included in this book are clean and natural. You can feel really good about what you are putting on and into your body. Your skin will thank you for it!

Enjoy that glow!

MORE BOOKS FROM JOSEPHINE SIMON

Homemade Bath Bombs and Bubble Baths

Learn to make your own All-Natural Bath Bombs and Bubble Baths at Home today! It's fun and easy!

Bath bombs and bubble bath make bath time so much more fun and enjoyable for adults and kids alike. The best part is that you can make your own at home. It's that easy. Relax in a luxurious hot bath of bubble and fizzies, rejuvenating and pampering your body, and awakening all your sense.

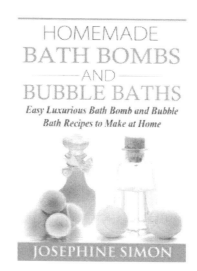

Essential Oils and Aromatherapy: A Beginner's Guide to Making and Using Essential Oils at Home for Skincare and Beauty Products

Want to revamp your beauty routine with all-natural beauty products you can make at home and gain a better knowledge of essential oils and aromatherapy?

Then this is the book for you! It will go through all the benefits and applications of essential oils in your daily routine. Essential oils are the most cost efficient and natural way to apply to your skin or for certain ailments. They can be used on multiple skin types to cure anything from lack of hydration to dealing with pesky facial acne or smoothing out wrinkles.

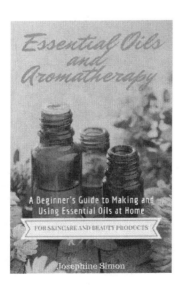